GASTRIC SLEEVE SURGERY MEAL PLAN

Comprehensive Guide Unlocking The Secrets
of nutrition after Surgery Success, Nourishing
Meal Plans, Recipes And Practical Tips For
Optimal Health And Wellness)

DR. ALLAN FREDA

Contents

CHAPTER 1 5

UNDERSTANDING GASTROINTESTINAL SLEEVE
SURGERY...7

CHAPTER 2 17

NAVIGATING DIETARY CHANGES........................17

CHAPTER 3 23

INGREDIENTS AND ESSENTIAL KITCHEN TOOLS
FOR BUILDING A FOUNDATION 23

CHAPTER 4..32

CREATING SCRUMPTIOUS AND NUTRITIOUS
BREAKFASTS 32

CHAPTER 5 37

APPEALABLE LUNCHES FOR IDEAL NUTRITION 37

CHAPTER 6..43

YUMMY DINNER RECIPES FOR PATIENTS WITH
GASTRIC SLEEVE DISEASES................................43

CHAPTER 7 48

SNACK TIME SOLUTIONS: HEALTHY TREATS IN-
BETWEEN MEALS 48

CHAPTER 8 54

DELICIOUS DEVICES WITHOUT RUNNING AWAY
FROM YOUR PROGRESS 54

CHAPTER 9 60

WEEKLY MENUS AND PREP TIPS FOR EASY MEAL
PLANNING 60

CHAPTER 10 70

MANAGING SOCIAL SETTLEMENTS AND
EXECUTING MENU 70

CONCLUSION 74

CONCERNING THIS BOOK

This book provides a thorough approach to managing the dietary adjustments required following gastric sleeve surgery. It gives recently diagnosed patients a thorough understanding of post-surgery nutrition and includes therapeutic recipes, meal planning, and professional advice for long-term well-being.

With the help of the book, readers should be able to optimize their diet following surgery and make sure they are getting all the nutrients they require to heal and stay healthy.

Through tried-and-true methods and useful guidance, this tool helps patients adjust to their new dietary needs, ensuring a seamless recovery and favorable long-term results after gastric sleeve surgery.

Disclaimer

The information in this book is for informational purposes only and should not replace professional medical advice, diagnosis, or treatment. Always consult your physician or a qualified health provider regarding any medical concerns. Do not disregard professional medical advice or delay seeking it based on information in this book.

The author does not endorse or have affiliations with any mentioned entities. References are for informational purposes only.

Consult your healthcare provider before making dietary or lifestyle changes, especially during recovery from surgery, as individual needs vary.

Results may vary, and the information provided is not guaranteed to produce specific outcomes.

By reading this book, you acknowledge and agree to consult your healthcare provider before implementing any information herein.

For further guidance, consult your healthcare provider or reputable medical websites for reliable information on surgery recovery diets.

CHAPTER 1

UNDERSTANDING GASTROINTESTINAL SLEEVE SURGERY

By shrinking the stomach, gastric sleeve surgery, commonly referred to as sleeve gastrectomy, is a surgical technique intended to facilitate weight loss. The stomach is severely reduced during this limiting operation, leaving just a tiny "sleeve" or tube-shaped stomach. Because of this change in the structure of the stomach, less food can be eaten, which reduces hunger and makes smaller meals feel fuller. When someone is extremely obese and has not been able to reduce weight with diet and exercise alone, gastric sleeve surgery is frequently advised. To make an informed decision about having gastric sleeve surgery, one must be aware of all the details surrounding the process, including its overview, risks and advantages, preparation, and post-surgical recovery.

A minimally invasive method that has gained popularity as an efficient treatment for obesity and accompanying medical issues is gastric sleeve surgery. About 75–80% of the stomach is removed by the surgeon during the procedure, leaving behind a smaller, pouch-shaped stomach.

Because of the reduced capacity of the stomach pouch, less food can be eaten, which results in a decrease in caloric intake and weight reduction. Because the intestines are not rerouted with gastric sleeve surgery, there may be fewer problems and nutritional deficits than with gastric bypass surgery. Furthermore, the process does not call for the insertion of an external device, like a gastric band. Compared to open surgery, gastric sleeve surgery is usually conducted laparoscopically, utilizing tiny incisions and a camera-guided scope, which shortens hospital stays and expedites recovery.

Advantages and Dangers

There are several possible advantages to gastric sleeve surgery for people who are battling with obesity and the health problems that come with it. Significant and long-lasting weight loss is one of the main advantages, as it can enhance general health and lower the risk of obesity-related diseases like type 2 diabetes, hypertension, and sleep apnea. Additionally, mobility, self-esteem, and quality of life may all improve as a result of weight loss following gastric sleeve surgery.

The long-term problems and risk of nutritional deficits associated with gastric sleeve surgery are generally lower than those of other bariatric surgeries like gastric bypass or gastric banding. However, there are some risks and potential consequences associated with gastric sleeve surgery, just like with other surgical operations.

These could include anesthesia-related side effects, bleeding, clotting, infection, and leaking from the surgical site. Before undergoing the treatment, patients thinking about gastric sleeve surgery should carefully examine their alternatives and discuss any potential risks and advantages with their healthcare professionals.

Getting Ready for Surgery

There are multiple phases involved in preparing for gastric sleeve surgery to maximize results and reduce problems. Patients will get a thorough medical examination before surgery to determine their general health status and fitness for the treatment. Blood tests, imaging studies, and consultations with a variety of medical specialists, including a psychologist, dietician, and surgeon, may be part of this examination.

Patients may be instructed to adhere to a preoperative diet in the weeks preceding surgery to minimize surgical risks and shrink the size of the liver.

To encourage weight loss and shrink the liver, this diet usually entails taking low-calorie, high-protein meal replacements or a liquid diet. Patients may also be advised to change their lifestyles to include things like upping physical activity, stopping smoking, and taking care of any underlying medical concerns. A successful surgery and the best possible results depend on careful planning and following preoperative instructions.

The Recovery After Surgery

A crucial part of the gastric sleeve surgery process is the post-surgical recovery phase, which calls for close attention to dietary recommendations, lifestyle modifications, and aftercare. Patients will have a brief hospital stay for monitoring and pain management right after surgery. They will progressively go from a clear liquid diet to a complete liquid diet throughout this phase, and if they can handle it, they will eventually switch to soft foods and solid foods. To avoid complications including vomiting, dumping syndrome, and dehydration, patients must adhere to their surgeon's advice regarding dietary progression, portion sizes, and frequency of meals.

Patients will be urged to include regular physical exercise in their daily routine in addition to dietary adjustments to assist in weight loss and enhance overall health.

It is crucial to schedule routine follow-up visits with the surgical team, which consists of the surgeon, dietician, and other medical specialists, to track recovery, handle any issues or difficulties, and offer continuing support and direction. Maintaining a balanced diet, engaging in regular exercise, and keeping up with follow-up appointments are all necessary for long-term success after gastric sleeve surgery in terms of weight loss and general well-being.

Adopting a healthy, balanced diet is crucial after gastric sleeve surgery to assist weight loss, encourage recovery, and ensure long-term success. A thorough post-operative food plan should prioritize meeting nutritional needs, reducing the chance of problems, and optimizing weight reduction results. The main ideas of a post-surgery diet will be covered in this guide, along with suggestions for foods, serving sizes, meal planning assistance, and professional counsel for long-term wellness.

Recipes and Meal Plans for Healing

Patients will follow a stepwise diet progression plan in the early post-surgery recovery phases, beginning with clear liquids and working their way up to solid foods over a few weeks. To avoid dehydration and facilitate recovery, the first phase emphasizes the consumption of clear liquids such as broth, sugar-free gelatin, and diluted fruit juices. Patients will be introduced to pureed foods, soft foods, and finally solid foods as tolerated as they go on to the following phases of the diet.

To assist healing, muscle maintenance, and weight loss, it is imperative to concentrate on ingesting nutrient-dense foods that are high in protein, vitamins, and minerals. Lean protein sources including fish, chicken, tofu, and beans can be included in meals to assist increase satiety and stop muscle loss when losing weight. Including a range of vibrant fruits and vegetables in meals can also supply vital vitamins, antioxidants, and fiber to promote digestive health and general well-being. A good post-surgery diet must include meal planning and preparation since they can keep patients on track with their nutritional objectives and reduce their dependency on processed or convenience meals. Incorporating a range of flavors and textures into meal planning while maintaining a balanced intake of lean protein, healthy fats, complex carbs, and fiber-rich foods can help patients achieve their dietary goals.

Mealtime can be made more fun and fulfilling by experimenting with healing dishes that include nutrient-dense foods and tasty herbs and spices. Personalized advice and help for creating a post-surgery meal plan that satisfies specific dietary choices, nutritional needs, and weight loss objectives can be obtained by working with a licensed dietitian or nutritionist.

Professional Advice for Long-Term Health

Long-term success after gastric sleeve surgery can be supported by implementing lifestyle modifications and self-care techniques into daily living in addition to adhering to a balanced diet. Maintaining muscle mass, encouraging weight loss, and enhancing general health and well-being all depend on regular physical activity.

Patients can keep active, feel more energized, and experience less stress by taking part in exercises like walking, swimming, cycling, or strength training. Making it a priority to stay well hydrated throughout the day by consuming lots of water can aid in digestion, encourage fullness, and prevent dehydration. Furthermore, mindful eating practices that involve chewing food carefully, enjoying every bite, and being aware of cues from hunger and fullness can assist patients in creating a positive relationship with food and avoiding overindulging. Throughout the post-surgery journey, establishing a strong support network of family, friends, and medical professionals can offer motivation, accountability, and direction.

It is imperative to attend routine follow-up sessions with the surgical team, which consists of the surgeon, nutritionist, and other medical professionals, to track recovery, address any issues or complications, and modify treatment plans as necessary. Through the implementation of a comprehensive post-surgical care plan that incorporates a wholesome diet, consistent exercise, and psychological assistance, patients can attain sustainable weight loss outcomes and enhance their general well-being and standard of living.

CHAPTER 2
NAVIGATING DIETARY CHANGES

Surgically removing a significant piece of the stomach to create a smaller stomach pouch that resembles a sleeve or tube is known as gastric sleeve surgery or sleeve gastrectomy. By lowering the stomach's capacity, this procedure helps obese people lose a large amount of weight. But to guarantee the best possible recovery and long-term weight control after gastric sleeve surgery, a significant food and lifestyle change is necessary. The creation and implementation of a healthy meal plan that is adapted to fulfill nutritional requirements and facilitate recovery after surgery is an essential component of this adjustment.

The Value of a Well-Designed Meal Plan:

Following gastric sleeve surgery, a healthy food plan is essential for stimulating weight loss, aiding with the healing process, and enhancing general health and wellness. Post-surgery, with a smaller stomach and changed digestive capacity, it is critical to limit calorie intake and prioritize nutrient-dense foods that include important vitamins, minerals, and protein.

A carefully thought-out meal plan encourages people to choose better foods, control portion sizes, and stay properly hydrated, all of which contribute to maximum nutrient absorption and maintained energy levels. A planned meal plan also gives people a sense of stability and control, which lowers the risk of overindulging or giving in to bad eating habits, which could compromise the results of the surgery.

Dietary Recommendations and Guidelines:
Patients usually follow certain dietary advice and limitations after gastric sleeve surgery to promote

recovery, avoid problems, and achieve good weight loss outcomes. People are initially put on a liquid or pureed diet to give their stomachs time to recover and become used to their smaller size. Clear liquids, protein shakes, and strained soups are the staples of this phase, which is followed by a gradual transition to thicker liquids and soft foods as tolerated.

Patients can gradually switch to a solid food diet, avoiding high-calorie, high-fat, and sugary foods and concentrating on lean protein sources, non-starchy vegetables, fruits, and whole grains. As the lower stomach capacity may limit food consumption, it is imperative to prioritize protein intake to support muscle preservation, enhance satiety, and prevent nutritional deficits.

People are also told to stay away from fizzy drinks, tough meats, fibrous foods, and foods heavy in sugar or fat since they can make it difficult to lose weight, induce dumping syndrome, or create pain.

A post-gastric sleeve surgery meal plan that works must emphasize portion control because the smaller stomach size limits the quantity of food that can be eaten at once. By putting portion control techniques into practice, people can better regulate how much food they consume, avoid overindulging, and increase satiety while still getting enough nutrients. Focusing on smaller, more frequent meals spaced evenly throughout the day to avoid undue stretching of the stomach pouch is one useful tactic.

Eating a diet high in protein and putting non-starchy veggies on half of the plate will help you construct balanced meals that are low in calories and high in nutrients. To prevent discomfort and encourage the best possible digestion, it's also essential to chew food well, eat slowly, and pay attention to your body's signals of hunger and fullness. Furthermore, the use of smaller bowls, plates, and cutlery might visually deceive the brain into thinking that there are greater servings, encouraging feelings of contentment without going overboard.

Managing Nutritional Requirements:

To assist healing, encourage weight reduction, and prevent nutritional deficits, a post-gastric sleeve surgery meal plan must achieve a balance of necessary elements. Since it is essential for maintaining muscle mass, accelerating the healing of wounds, and maintaining metabolic processes, protein continues to be a fundamental food.

To satisfy protein needs and encourage fullness, lean protein sources including fish, poultry, eggs, tofu, lentils, and low-fat dairy products ought to be given priority at each meal. A well-rounded diet that includes vital vitamins, minerals, fiber, and antioxidants is also ensured by including a range of nutrient-dense foods, such as fruits, vegetables, whole grains, and healthy fats.

To create a personalized meal plan that satisfies dietary restrictions, addresses individual nutritional needs, and promotes long-term wellness, it is imperative to collaborate with a certified dietitian or other healthcare professional. To avoid deficiencies and improve health outcomes, regular monitoring of nutrient levels by blood testing and supplements may be required.

To assist healing, encourage weight reduction, and guarantee long-term success, managing dietary changes following gastric sleeve surgery calls for meticulous planning, attention to dietary guidelines, and an emphasis on nutrient-dense meals.

A well-crafted meal plan that is customized to each person's demands, tastes, and dietary needs acts as a guide for choosing better foods, controlling portion sizes, and regaining optimal health and wellness after surgery. After having gastric sleeve surgery, people can improve their quality of life, vigor, and health by managing their nutritional requirements, according to dietary guidelines, and using portion management techniques.

CHAPTER 3

INGREDIENTS AND ESSENTIAL KITCHEN TOOLS FOR BUILDING A FOUNDATION

Setting out on a path to maximum health after gastric sleeve surgery requires careful consideration of food choices. Having a well-stocked kitchen and a thorough understanding of the necessary ingredients are crucial to this endeavor.

Having the correct equipment and supplies on hand can make meal preparation after surgery much easier, regardless of experience level or inexperience with cooking.

This part will explore essential kitchen tools, basic items for meal prep using gastric sleeves, and priceless advice on smart grocery shopping, providing a strong basis for your culinary pursuits.

Important kitchen appliances

Purchasing the right kitchenware is essential to carrying out a gastric sleeve meal plan effectively.

A few essential instruments are essential for meal preparation following surgery, while the specifics may differ depending on individual preferences and cooking techniques. To begin with, having a trustworthy set of sharp knives is crucial for accurately dicing, slicing, and cutting items. Choosing top-notch knives not only improves safety but also simplifies food preparation.

It's also essential to stock your kitchen with multipurpose cookware, such as baking sheets, pans, and pots. Particularly useful for reducing the need for unnecessary cooking oils and encouraging healthier meal options are non-stick models.

A sturdy food processor or blender is a great tool for pureeing vegetables and adding healthy components to smoothies, soups, and sauces. Additionally, purchasing a digital kitchen scale allows for precise portion control, making it easier to follow suggested serving sizes.

In addition, you might want to equip your kitchen with useful tools like a mandoline slicer for consistent fruit and vegetable slicing and a vegetable spiralizer for creating creative low-carb alternatives. These are not necessary, but they can improve your cooking skills and provide your post-surgery menu with some variation.

Essential Components for Preparing Gastric Sleeve Meals

Creating a comprehensive pantry is necessary to carry out a gastric sleeve food plan effectively. It is critical to prioritize nutrient-dense, high-protein diets while reducing processed carbohydrates and fats to enhance post-surgery healing and advance long-term health. Prioritize the following basic supplies when restocking your kitchen:

Lean Protein Sources: To assist muscle maintenance after surgery and to promote satiety, include lean protein sources such as skinless chicken, fish, tofu, lentils, and eggs in your meal plan. Choose baked, poached, or grilled recipes to maximize flavor and reduce additional fats.

Fresh Produce: Stuff your face with a rainbow of vibrant fruits and veggies to add vital vitamins, minerals, and antioxidants to your food. Particularly nutrient-rich foods include berries, citrus fruits, leafy greens, cruciferous vegetables, and tomatoes. To keep your meals interesting and fulfilling, try including a range of textures and flavors.

Whole Grains and Complex Carbohydrates: Consuming whole grains and complex carbohydrates in moderation can give prolonged energy and dietary fiber, even if carbohydrate consumption should be restricted after surgery. Quinoa, whole wheat products, barley, oats, and brown rice are great options for supporting digestive health and controlling blood sugar levels.

Healthy Fats: Although fats should be eaten in moderation, adding foods high in healthy fats, including avocados, nuts, seeds, and olive oil, can provide important nutrients and increase fullness. For best heart health, use minimally and give unsaturated fats priority over saturated and trans fats.

Low-Fat Dairy or Dairy Alternatives: To promote bone health and supply vital minerals, choose low-fat dairy products or dairy alternatives fortified with calcium and vitamin D. Dairy products without a lot of fat can be included in your diet plan with Greek yogurt, skim milk, almond milk, and fortified soy products.

Stocking up on pantry essentials like whole grain pasta, low-sodium broths, canned beans, and herbs and spices can also improve the taste and adaptability of your meals without sacrificing their nutritional value.

Advice for Savvy Purchasing

Using your discernment when navigating grocery store aisles is essential to following a gastric sleeve meal plan and maximizing nutrition after surgery. By using these smart shopping guidelines, you may prioritize nutrient-dense foods and make well-informed decisions when you shop:

Plan Ahead: Make a thorough shopping list, check your weekly meal plan, and assess your pantry before you go to the grocery store. Making a list helps you avoid impulsive purchases and guarantees that you have everything you need to make wholesome meals.

Shop the Periphery: Fresh produce, lean meats, dairy goods, and whole grains are usually found at the periphery of the supermarket. By concentrating your shopping efforts in these locations, you can minimize your exposure to highly processed snacks and sugary beverages in the center aisles and prioritize whole, less processed foods.

Read Nutrition Labels Carefully: Pay close attention to serving sizes, total calories, protein content, added sugars, and unwanted ingredients like trans fats and high salt when choosing packaged goods.

Choose items with identifiable, whole-food ingredients and shorter ingredient lists.

Select Frozen and Canned Types: Although fresh food is the best option, frozen and canned fruits and vegetables can be useful substitutes, especially for produce that is out of season or when time is of the essence.

Select alternatives free of added sweeteners, syrups, or high sodium content.

To further lower the salt amount, rinse canned veggies.

Think About Purchasing in Bulk: Purchasing some basics in large quantities, such as grains, legumes, nuts, and seeds, can save money and reduce packaging waste.

To preserve freshness and make sure bulk ingredients are always available for meal preparation, store them in airtight containers.

Emphasise Quality Over Quantity: Although financial constraints should be taken into account, whenever feasible, give top priority to purchasing nutrient-dense, high-quality foods.

Choose sustainably farmed seafood, organic fruit, and grass-fed meats to reduce your exposure to hormones, pesticides, and other environmental toxins.

You may optimize your shopping efficiency, maximize the nutritional content of your purchases, and maintain compliance with your post-surgery dietary objectives by utilizing these techniques.

The first step in creating a successful post-gastric sleeve surgery meal plan is putting together the required cooking equipment and storing up key items. It is possible to empower oneself to cook nourishing and delicious meals that support your long-term health and wellness journey by buying wisely, investing in high-quality equipment, and giving priority to foods high in nutrients.

CHAPTER 4
CREATING SCRUMPTIOUS AND NUTRITIOUS BREAKFASTS

Breakfast is frequently seen as the most significant meal of the day, and those who have had gastric sleeve surgery may find this to be especially true.

A nutritious breakfast not only speeds up your metabolism but also establishes the pattern of your eating throughout the day. It's important to customize your breakfast options after gastric sleeve surgery to make sure they're not just tasty but also full of the vital nutrients your body needs to recover and thrive. We will look at a variety of breakfast options in our in-depth guide to the post-surgery diet, with an emphasis on protein-rich options, energizing options, and quick yet healthy meals to help you start your day off well.

It's critical to make breakfast choices following gastric sleeve surgery that support recovery and provide you with consistent energy throughout the morning.

Muesli and whole wheat bread are two examples of whole grains that provide a great base for breakfast because they include complex carbs that release energy gradually and keep you feeling full and energized.

These can be used with lean protein sources like eggs, Greek yogurt, or turkey bacon to increase the nutritious content of your breakfast and increase satiety. Incorporating fresh fruits, like bananas or berries, into your morning meal will also naturally sweeten it and provide some vitamins and minerals.

Smoothies with high-protein components, such as protein powder, spinach, and almond milk, can also be a quick and energizing choice, particularly for people with hectic schedules.

Protein is a vital part of a post-surgery diet since it is necessary for muscle growth and tissue regeneration. Breakfasting on meals high in protein can support long-term weight management objectives and aid in the healing process.

Whether they are poached, scrambled, or combined with veggies to make an omelet, eggs are a healthy and adaptable option.

Greek yogurt is another great source of protein; in addition to providing necessary amino acids, it also contains probiotics that assist digestive health.

To increase the protein level of breakfast meals, lean chicken or fish cuts, cottage cheese, and tofu can be added. If you are looking for plant-based solutions, you can still get enough protein from your morning meal by adding things like quinoa, chia seeds, or hemp hearts.

They also offer flavour and texture.

Simple and Quick Breakfast Ideas:

It might be difficult to find time in the daily shuffle to make a healthy breakfast. But, you may prepare quick and simple breakfast dishes that satisfy your dietary requirements after surgery with a little forethought and ingenuity.

A quick and easy option, overnight oats may be made the night before and personalized with different toppings like fruit, nuts, and seeds for extra taste and nutrients. Making portable breakfast choices, like protein bars or muffins with nutritious grains and protein powder, can also help with hectic mornings.

Furthermore, preparing materials ahead of time— for example, by cutting vegetables or pre-cooking eggs—can speed up the breakfast preparation process and increase the availability of healthy options throughout the workweek.

After gastric sleeve surgery, you can support your recovery and long-term wellness objectives by making nutrient-dense ingredients a priority and combining them into simple yet fulfilling breakfast recipes. This will help you start your mornings off right.

CHAPTER 5

APPEALABLE LUNCHES FOR IDEAL NUTRITION

Lunches that satisfy are essential for sustaining appropriate nutrition after gastric sleeve surgery. Feeding the body nutritional meals that promote healing and general well-being is crucial as it heals and adapts to its increased digestive capacity. Including a range of nutrient-dense foods in lunch meals not only helps satisfy daily dietary requirements but also increases energy and satiety levels for the day. This section will explore three types of filling lunches that are appropriate for those who have had gastric sleeve surgery: Hearty Soup and Sandwich Combos, Portable Lunches for Busy Days, and Wholesome Salad Creations.

Healthy Salad Recipes: With so many different nutrients and tastes available in one dish, salads are a flexible choice for lunches following surgery.

Incorporating lean proteins, vibrant veggies, healthy fats, and fiber-rich components is crucial when creating salads for people recuperating from gastric sleeve surgery. Protein foods that include the essential amino acids needed for muscle maintenance and tissue regeneration include canned tuna, grilled chicken, turkey breast, and tofu. Adding leafy greens as a basis, such as kale, spinach, or mixed lettuces, also adds nutrition and volume without adding extra calories.

In addition to adding visual appeal, colorful vegetables like bell peppers, cucumbers, cherry tomatoes, and shredded carrots also include vitamins, minerals, and antioxidants that are essential for the immune system and healing. Avocado slices, almonds, seeds, or a drizzle of olive oil can all help to provide flavor and healthful fats. To limit calorie intake and encourage weight reduction, stay away from high-calorie toppings like bacon bits, croutons, and creamy dressings. Alternatively, make your vinaigrettes with simple, low-fat, or low-sugar components like lemon juice, balsamic vinegar, Dijon mustard, and herbs for flavor.

Warm Soup and Sandwich Sets: For those recuperating from gastric sleeve surgery, soup and sandwiches provide a nourishing and filling lunch choice. To cut down on extra fat and calories, choose pureed or broth-based soups rather than creamy or heavier ones.

Soups containing lean proteins, such as fish, poultry, or lentils, can boost satiety and supply vital nutrients. Vegetables such as carrots, celery, onions, and leafy greens offer vitamins, minerals, and fiber to the meal. Whole-grain bread or wraps are a good choice for sandwiches because they are high in dietary fiber and complex carbs, which help with digestion and blood sugar regulation.

The main course can be lean protein options such as grilled chicken, roast beef, hummus, or sliced turkey.

Adding lettuce, tomato, cucumber, and other vegetables improves the dish's flavor and nutritional content. Condiments that are low in fat and calories, such as salsa, mustard, and Greek yogurt-based spreads, can be used to enhance flavour and moisture. Furthermore, adding avocado slices or low-fat cheese can give extra nutrients and a creamy mouthfeel. A small wrap or half-sandwich goes well with a cup of soup to help with portion management and fulfill hunger and nutritional needs.

Lunch Ideas That Are Portable for Busy Days: Those with hectic schedules need to consider lunch options that are portable to maintain their post-surgery dietary objectives. Making nutrient-rich grab-and-go meals in advance can assist avoid making rash food decisions and guarantee that they are always available. Focus on putting together balanced meals with a mix of protein, carbs, healthy fats, and fiber when organizing carry-along lunches. Meal prep ideas such as compartmentalized containers or bento box-style meals can help with portion management and keeping food distinct until lunchtime. Convenient major components can be protein-rich foods like Greek yogurt cups, hard-boiled eggs, chicken or turkey skewers, or protein bars. Protein and whole-food carbohydrates, such as quinoa salad cups, fruit slices, vegetable sticks, and whole-grain crackers, work well together to offer sustained energy and encourage satiety.

Incorporating wholesome fats from foods like olives, nuts, seeds, and avocados enhances flavor and prevents hunger. Perishable foods can also be kept fresh and safe to eat all day by placing an ice pack inside a small cooler bag. People can keep a healthy eating habit even on busy days by organizing and prepping their portable lunches.

Nutrient density, quantity control, and meal variety are important considerations when creating satiating lunches for optimal nutrition following gastric sleeve surgery.

A balanced diet that includes lean proteins, vibrant veggies, whole grains, healthy fats, and foods high in fiber can help people achieve their long-term wellness and recuperation objectives. Prioritizing nutrient-rich ingredients and thoughtful eating practices can help people thrive on their post-surgery path, whether they are enjoying healthy salad concoctions, robust soup and sandwich combos, or portable lunches for busy days.

CHAPTER 6

YUMMY DINNER RECIPES FOR PATIENTS WITH GASTRIC SLEEVE DISEASES

By reducing the size of the stomach, gastric sleeve surgery, sometimes referred to as sleeve gastrectomy, helps patients lose weight by limiting the quantity of food they may eat. Patients must follow a balanced diet after this procedure to promote healthy recovery, ideal weight loss, and long-term well-being.

As one of the primary meals of the day, dinner has to be prepared with extra care to make sure it's wholesome and filling. We'll look at tasty supper recipes in this guide that are specially designed for those with gastric sleeves, with an emphasis on one-pot marvels that cook up quickly, vegetable-focused meals, and protein-rich entrees.

Rich in Protein Entrees:

For those having gastric sleeve surgery, protein is a vital nutrient since it helps with satiety, weight loss, and muscle restoration. Part of meal planning after surgery should be centered around protein-rich dishes. Choose lean protein sources including eggs, fish, poultry, and tofu.

A delectable and easy dinner option is grilled chicken breast seasoned with herbs and spices.

As an alternative, think about roasting salmon fillets and having them with steamed veggies on the side for a wholesome and satisfying dinner.

Add beans or tofu to salads or stir-fries for vegetarian options. Complete protein quinoa can also serve as the foundation for Buddha bowls topped with a tahini dressing and a variety of vegetables.

Try a variety of protein sources to ensure that your meals are enjoyable and diverse while yet satisfying your nutritional requirements.

Vegetable-Based Recipes:

Vegetables are a vital component of any gastric sleeve patient's diet since they are full of fiber, vitamins, and minerals. Including vegetable-focused dishes on dinner, menus improves the flavor and texture of meals while also adding nutritional value.

Roasted veggies with garlic, olive oil, and herbs make a flavorful side dish or may be served as a substantial main meal when paired with nutritious grains. For an eye-catching and filling supper alternative, try stuffing bell peppers with quinoa, black beans, corn, and salsa. "Zoodles," or zucchini noodles, are a low-carb substitute for classic pasta. They make a tasty and light dinner when served with grilled vegetables and marinara sauce.

Try a variety of vegetable combinations and cooking techniques to find new favorite foods that help you meet your post-surgery nutritional goals. Don't be afraid to try new things.

Hands-On Recipes for Easy Cooking:

When preparing meals after gastric sleeve surgery, ease of use and simplicity become crucial, particularly in the evenings when schedules are hectic. One-pot marvels provide a solution by making tasty, nourishing meals with little cleanup. One bowl full of healthful grains, veggies, and protein may be found in soups and stews, which make great one-pot meal options.

For a filling dinner that's easy on the stomach, try making a lentil stew that's packed with herbs and spices or a robust soup made with chicken and vegetables. For hectic weeknights, one-pot pasta meals like vegetable primavera with whole wheat noodles or spaghetti with turkey meatballs and marinara sauce are also easy and quick choices. Purchasing a pressure cooker or slow cooker might help you prepare meals even more easily since you can just set it and forget about it until suppertime. One-pot marvels are great for gastric sleeve patients who want convenience without losing flavor or nutrition since they allow you to have satisfying dinners without spending hours in the kitchen or worrying about unnecessary cleanup.

Creating mouthwatering supper recipes for people with gastric sleeves means emphasizing nutrient-dense foods, well-balanced macronutrients, and easy but tasty cooking techniques. In addition to supporting long-term well-being and post-surgery healing, protein-rich meals, vegetable-centric dishes, and one-pot marvels offer a variety of options to meet varied tastes and dietary requirements. During your gastric sleeve journey, you can have fulfilling dinners that support optimal health and weight loss by adding these recipes to your meal planning.

CHAPTER 7

SNACK TIME SOLUTIONS: HEALTHY TREATS IN-BETWEEN MEALS

When it comes to meal planning after gastric sleeve surgery, thoughtful snacks are essential for preserving energy levels, maximizing nutrient intake, and promoting the body's healing process. To guarantee a well-rounded dietary approach favorable to long-term health, this extensive book explores the fundamentals of wise snacking techniques, presents a variety of wholesome snack recipes catered to post-surgery demands and offers simple on-the-go snack ideas.

Clever Snacking Techniques

Following gastric sleeve surgery, it's critical to follow sensible snacking practices to increase fullness, reduce overindulgence during meals, and keep blood sugar levels stable.

Focusing on nutrient density and choosing snacks high in protein, vital minerals, and vitamins while watching portion sizes are some of the core ideas. Lean protein, good fats, and complex carbs are examples of macronutrients that should be included in a balanced diet to promote long-term energy release and healthy muscle building.

Additionally, limiting empty calories and maximizing nutritional content can be achieved by giving whole, minimally processed foods priority over sugary or high-calorie snacks. Furthermore, engaging in mindful eating practices, such as chewing deeply and appreciating every meal, improves enjoyment and builds a stronger bond with food, which lowers the probability of mindless snacking.

Successful snacking also involves planning and preparation because having healthy options on hand helps reduce impulsive purchases and encourage dietary adherence.

People can develop a healthy snacking habit that improves their general health and well-being by including these techniques in their post-surgery meal planning.

Healthy Snack Recipes

Creating wholesome snack recipes that are suited to the particular dietary needs following gastric sleeve surgery is essential to guaranteeing recovery and sufficient nourishment.

High-protein snack meals that include lean meats, Greek yogurt, or cottage cheese support the maintenance and repair of muscles while warding off hunger. Snacks high in protein include cottage cheese paired with sliced veggies, turkey and avocado roll-ups, and Greek yogurt parfaits topped with berries and almonds.

Nutrient absorption is facilitated and vital fatty acids are supplied when snacks contain sources of healthy fats like avocado, almonds, and seeds.

Nut butter on apple slices, guacamole with whole-grain crackers, or a handful of mixed nuts are healthy choices high in good fats. Including whole grains, fruits, and vegetables high in fiber in snack recipes also helps to maintain healthy digestion and control blood sugar levels.

Some examples are whole-grain toast with mashed avocado and cherry tomatoes, carrot sticks with hummus, or a small apple with nut butter. Individuals can create delicious snack options that meet their post-surgery nutritional objectives and promote optimal healing and recovery by experimenting with a variety of nutrient-dense products and flavors.

Quick and Easy Snack Ideas

After gastric sleeve surgery, managing hectic lifestyles and busy schedules calls for portable, simple-to-make, and nutritionally balanced on-the-go snack alternatives. When you portion out snacks in advance and store them in resealable bags or grab-and-go containers, you can avoid making impulsive food decisions when you're out and about. Protein-dense foods like turkey jerky, string cheese, and hard-boiled eggs are quick and easy ways to get satisfying protein when you're on the road. When time is limited and you're having a hectic day, snack bars containing whole food ingredients like nuts, seeds, and dried fruits are a simple answer.

Choosing pre-cut veggies and single-serve hummus or Greek yogurt dip makes for a nutrient-rich, hydrating snack that tastes good anytime, anywhere. Furthermore, having a supply of transportable fruits on hand, like apples, bananas, or grapes, guarantees a quick and wholesome snack choice for when hunger hits while out and about. People can easily add on-the-go snacks into their post-surgery meal plan, supporting their long-term wellness goals while managing their busy lifestyles, by prioritizing convenience without sacrificing nutritional quality.

To achieve and maintain maximum health and well-being after gastric sleeve surgery, it is imperative to learn the art of smart snacking. Through the implementation of tactical snacking techniques, exploration of wholesome snack recipes, and acceptance of portable, easily consumable snack concepts, people can develop a well-rounded and fulfilling nutritional regimen that facilitates their recovery process and promotes sustained achievement. Snack time may be a rewarding and satisfying component of the post-surgery meal plan, enabling people to flourish on their journey to wellness with careful planning, preparation, and an emphasis on nutrient density.

CHAPTER 8

DELICIOUS DEVICES WITHOUT RUNNING AWAY FROM YOUR PROGRESS

Desserts can still be enjoyed even after having gastric sleeve surgery. But it's important to make decisions that support your health objectives and correspond with your post-surgery dietary requirements. If you choose wisely and limit your intake, desserts can still be included in your meal plan. In this section, we'll look at a variety of dessert options that will help you lose weight and improve your general health in addition to satisfying your sweet tooth.

Sweet Treats Without Any Guilt:

Sweets with a hint of sweetness but no added sugar, bad fats, or excessive calories are guilt-free options that won't impede your recovery from gastric sleeve surgery.

Because they are usually produced with simple, healthful ingredients and minimal processing, these sweets are sure to satisfy your cravings without interfering with your weight loss attempts.

This includes options like homemade fruit sorbets, sugar-free gelatin, and Greek yogurt parfaits topped with fresh berries.

In addition to being incredibly tasty, these desserts please your palate and don't violate any of your dietary requirements.

It's important to consider ingredients and portion quantities while choosing guilt-free sweets. Desserts high in fiber and low in added sugars are better choices since they can help you control your blood sugar levels while still feeling full and content.

To further improve the nutritional value of your desserts and aid in satiety and muscular recovery after surgery, try adding protein-rich items like almonds or Greek yogurt.

Desserts with Fruit:

Fruits are a natural sweetener and make a great dessert for anyone on a post-gastric sleeve surgery food plan. Fruits are inherently sweet and tasty, but they are also a great source of important vitamins, minerals, and antioxidants that promote general health and well-being. Adding a range of fruits to your dessert selections will enhance their color, flavor, and nutritional content without making it harder to reach your weight loss objectives.

Fruit salads, fruit skewers with yogurt dip, and baked fruit crisps with oats and almonds are a few common fruit-based dessert alternatives.

These desserts include vital nutrients that aid in healing and recuperation following surgery, and they have the ideal ratio of sweetness to texture. Fruits high in vitamin C, such as kiwis, oranges, and berries, can also strengthen your immune system and promote wound healing, which is a crucial part of the recuperation process following surgery.

To optimize nutritional diversity and flavor in fruit-based sweets, try to use a range of fruits.

Try a variety of combos and presentation techniques to keep your dinners interesting and fun. Fruit-based desserts can be eaten on their own or combined with a protein-rich side dish like cottage cheese or Greek yogurt to satisfy your sweet taste and advance your long-term wellness objectives.

Recipes for decadent but sensible desserts:

After gastric sleeve surgery, it may seem paradoxical to indulge in rich, indulgent sweets, but it is still possible to occasionally indulge in delights in moderation and with awareness. Dessert dishes that are decadent but sensible are those that provide a hint of luxury without interfering with your diet or your efforts to lose weight.

Because these treats are usually prepared with healthy ingredients and in appropriate sizes, you can indulge your cravings without sacrificing your long-term health objectives.

Desserts such as avocado chocolate mousse, baked oatmeal cookies, and dark chocolate-dipped strawberries are decadent but healthy options that can be consumed in moderation after surgery. These sweet treats offer a fulfilling treat along with health advantages like fiber, antioxidants, and heart-healthy lipids.

You can occasionally indulge in sweets without feeling guilty or suffering unfavorable effects if you make dessert selections that emphasize high-quality ingredients and amount control.

Portion control and attentive eating are crucial when including rich but moderate dessert recipes in your meal plan. To avoid overindulging, savor every bite and pay attention to your body's signals of hunger and fullness. Additionally, to assist control blood sugar levels and encourage satiety, think about including dessert in a balanced meal. Overindulgent desserts can be enjoyed occasionally without deviating from your post-surgery dietary requirements and long-term wellness objectives if you approach them mindfully and in moderation.

CHAPTER 9
WEEKLY MENUS AND PREP TIPS FOR EASY MEAL PLANNING

Planning your meals is essential to keeping up a healthy lifestyle, especially after having gastric sleeve surgery. Patients must follow an organized nutrition plan after surgery to facilitate weight loss, speed healing, and avoid problems.

With its extensive menu planning, therapeutic recipes, and professional advice for long-term wellness, this comprehensive guide seeks to offer insights into creating the ideal post-surgery diet. Through an emphasis on methodical meal planning, weekly menu samples, and batch cooking techniques, people can streamline the process of following dietary rules and facilitate a seamless shift towards a better way of living.

Planning meals effectively starts with being aware of the dietary restrictions and requirements after gastric sleeve surgery. Post-operative diets usually involve multiple stages, beginning with clear liquids and progressively moving on to pureed, soft, and then solid foods. A qualified dietician or healthcare expert should be consulted to identify the proper course of action and customize the meal plan to meet the needs of each individual.

To begin meal planning, make a list of foods that are allowed at each stage of the diet. Lean meats, chicken, fish, eggs, and plant-based proteins like tofu and beans should all be on this list of protein sources. A balanced nutrient intake is also guaranteed by including a range of fruits, vegetables, whole grains, and healthy fats. Portion management is essential to avoid discomfort and promote healthy digestion, particularly in the early phases of recovery.

Making a weekly meal plan comes next after the list of permitted items is finalized. This entails choosing dishes that incorporate a balance of macronutrients and micronutrients and comply with dietary standards. A source of protein, carbs, and good fats should be included in every meal, along with lots of water to stay hydrated. Smaller, more frequent meals spread out throughout the day are a good way to encourage satiety and avoid overindulging.

Weekly Menu Samples

Weekly menu samples offer a workable structure for carrying out the meal plan and guaranteeing diversity in each day's meal. You can alter these recipes to suit your dietary requirements, nutritional requirements, and personal tastes.

This is an example of a weekly menu that someone on the post-gastric sleeve surgery diet might follow:

Monday

- Greek yogurt topped with berries and almonds for breakfast

- Snack: A protein shake with a banana and unsweetened almond milk

- Lunch would be grilled chicken salad topped with cherry tomatoes, mixed greens, and balsamic vinaigrette.

- Snack: Hummus-topped carrot sticks

- Supper is baked salmon over quinoa and steamed broccoli.

Tuesday

- Whole grain bread and scrambled eggs with spinach for breakfast

- Snack: Pineapple chunks mixed with cottage cheese

- Turkey lettuce wraps with salsa and avocado for lunch

• Snack: walnuts and honey paired with Greek yogurt

• Dinner is brown rice and stir-fried tofu with mixed veggies.

Wednesday

• Smoothie for breakfast consisting of almond milk, spinach, banana, and protein powder

• Snack: Peanut butter-topped apple slices

• Quinoa salad with cucumber, feta cheese and grilled prawns for lunch

• Snack: Mozzarella cheese and cherry tomatoes

• Dinner is cauliflower rice with a stir-fried dish of lean meat, onions, and bell peppers.

Thursday

• Muesli with sliced strawberries and honey drizzled over it for breakfast.

• Snack: Bar of protein

• Lean ground turkey and marinara sauce over zucchini noodles for lunch

• Snack: Slices of peach and cottage cheese

• Supper is grilled pork chops along with green beans and roasted sweet potatoes.

Friday

• Whole grain cereal, skim milk, and sliced bananas for breakfast

• Snack: Trail mix flavored with almonds and raisins

• Lunch would be whole grain toast and lentil soup.

• Edamame beans as a snack

• Supper is baked fish over quinoa pilaf and roasted Brussels sprouts.

On Saturday

• Egg muffins with feta cheese, tomatoes, and spinach for breakfast

• Snack: Granola and Greek yogurt

• Brown rice, stir-fried chicken, and vegetables for lunch.

• Snack: Cottage cheese and mixed fruit

• Dinner is couscous and grilled prawn skewers with grilled vegetables.

Sunday

• Pancakes made with whole grains, fresh berries, and maple syrup for breakfast.

• Snack: Banana and almond milk protein shake

• Lunch is a whole wheat tortilla with a turkey and avocado wrap.

• Snack: Peanut butter-covered celery sticks

• Supper consists of baked chicken breast over quinoa and roasted root vegetables.

A well-planned weekly menu, such as the one above, can help people make sure they're getting the nutrients they need while also eating a range of delectable and filling meals. It's critical to modify portion sizes in accordance with your protein and calorie needs, as recommended by medical experts.

Methods for Preparing Meals and Batch Cooking

Particularly for people with hectic schedules, batch cooking, and meal prep techniques simplify the meal planning process and make it simpler to follow nutritional recommendations.

Batch cooking is making big amounts of food ahead of time and freezing it for later use. This guarantees that wholesome foods are accessible when hunger strikes in addition to saving time.

Setting aside a day of the week, like Sunday, to prepare supplies and meals for the following week is an efficient way to batch cook. This could entail roasting a range of vegetables, cooking grains like quinoa or brown rice, and cooking proteins like chicken, fish, or tofu in large quantities. After cooking, these ingredients can be kept separately in the freezer or fridge for convenient access all week long.

Meal prep approaches, in addition to batch cooking, concentrate on putting together meals that are ready to eat and can be consumed cold or quickly reheated. This may be making salads to put in mason jars, putting up wraps or sandwiches, or setting out little snacks like hummus and chopped vegetables. People can resist the lure of harmful convenience foods and make sure they always have nutrient-dense options on hand by devoting a few hours of their week to meal prep.

It is critical to prioritize portion control and nutrient density during batch cooking and meal preparation for patients undergoing gastric sleeve surgery. An important component of aiding weight loss and general health is avoiding processed meals that are high in calories, fat, and sugar. Rather, give priority to entire meals that are high in fiber, lean protein, vitamins, and minerals to nourish the body and aid in healing.

Meal planning doesn't have to be difficult; it's an essential part of recovery from gastric sleeve surgery. People can easily navigate their post-surgery diet by using sample weekly menus, batch cooking and meal prep techniques, and a step-by-step meal planning guide. Long-term wellness and weight control objectives can be met with diligent preparation and commitment to wholesome eating practices.

CHAPTER 10
MANAGING SOCIAL SETTLEMENTS AND EXECUTING MENU

One important thing to think about when pursuing optimal health after gastric sleeve surgery is how to handle social situations and eating out.

These circumstances can be difficult since they can involve peer pressure, temptation, and the need to explain dietary restrictions. However, people can effectively handle these situations while adhering to their post-surgery diet plan and long-term wellness objectives with careful preparation, useful ideas, and open communication.

Techniques for Eating Out a Successfully

After gastric sleeve surgery, eating out calls for careful planning to maintain dietary restrictions while yet taking advantage of the social aspects of dining out.

A good approach is to do your homework on restaurants in advance and choose those that provide a good selection of healthful food and are open to unique requests. When looking through the menu, steer clear of fried or highly processed dishes and instead concentrate on lean proteins, veggies, and complete grains.

To further reduce unnecessary calories and regulate quantities, think about requesting meal adjustments, such as steamed vegetables in place of high-carb sides or the side order of sauces and dressings. To avoid pain and overeating, it is also helpful to adopt mindful eating practices, such as eating slowly, chewing food well, and stopping when you are comfortably satisfied.

Managing Get-togethers and Social Events

Food plays a major role in social events and get-togethers, which can make it difficult for people on a post-surgery diet plan.

It's crucial to discuss dietary requirements and preferences in advance with hosts or event organizers to handle these circumstances properly. By bringing food that fits your meal plan, you can guarantee that there will be something to eat. Redirecting attention from eating, concentrating on participating in activities or discussions that don't only revolve around food.

When attending potluck or buffet-style gatherings, consider all of your options before adding food to your plate. Give top priority to vegetables and meals high in protein, and restrict items high in calories and fat. Always pay attention to your body's signals of hunger and fullness, and stop eating when you're satisfied rather than consuming more food just because it's there.

Advice on Expressing Your Nutritional Requirements

After surgery, good communication is essential when dining out or going to social gatherings. When you communicate your dietary demands and limits clearly, people will be able to comprehend and meet your needs.

Don't be afraid to let waiters or restaurant employees know that you recently had gastric sleeve surgery and that your doctor has prescribed some dietary restrictions when you are dining out. When requesting menu item alterations or ingredient substitutions to suit your demands, be courteous but firm. Carrying a little card or note outlining your dietary restrictions might also be useful as it will facilitate communication with wait staff and chefs. Take the initiative to inform friends and family about your dietary limitations and the significance of following your meal plan for your health and well-being while you're in social situations like parties or get-togethers.

Through cultivating courteous and transparent communication, you may handle social circumstances with self-assurance and the assistance of others around you.

After gastric sleeve surgery, handling social settings and eating out calls for preparation, practical solutions, and honest communication.

People can stick to their post-surgery food plan while still enjoying social interactions and long-term health by putting ideas for dining out, navigating social events and gatherings, and effectively conveying their dietary needs into practice. People can overcome these obstacles and prosper on their path to better health and vitality if they are patient, persistent, and have the help of friends, family, and medical professionals.

CONCLUSION

Following gastric sleeve surgery, there is more that needs to be done to support healing and long-term wellness. It necessitates a comprehensive strategy that includes attentive decision-making, dietary modifications, and lifestyle alterations.

We have covered every facet of life after surgery in this extensive handbook, from comprehending the process to navigating the complex world of dietary adjustments. We've talked about how crucial it is to create a healthy meal plan, follow nutritional recommendations, and become proficient with portion management techniques.

By starting with the basic materials and cooking utensils, we've given ourselves the ability to make wholesome, delectable meals that are specifically catered to the needs of gastric sleeve patients.

Every recipe and recommendation, from hearty breakfast options to filling lunches and romantic dinners, has been carefully chosen to provide the best possible nutrition and healing.

We've also covered the difficulties associated with indulging and snacking, providing shrewd tactics and guilt-free dessert alternatives that permit enjoyment without impeding progress.

By making meal planning simple with tools like batch cooking and example menus, we've given people the confidence to take charge of their diets.

Beyond the kitchen, we've offered tips for interacting with others and going out to eat, making sure that people can satisfy their nutritional requirements without giving up on social interaction or enjoyment.

Essentially, this guide is about creating a sustainable lifestyle that supports long-term wellness and eases the transition into a new chapter of health and energy, not only about what to eat. People can start on a path to long-lasting wellness, healing, and growth by adopting the values presented in these pages and utilizing the power of nutrient-dense food.